Smoothie Recipes for Rapid Weight Loss

Table of Contents

Introduction

I want to thank and congratulate you for downloading the book *"Smoothie Recipes for Rapid Weight Loss"*.

It's a tough and busy life that people live these days but that does not mean that you should let yourself go and that you should not be concerned about your health. In fact, it should be your primary concern.

Losing weight is not just about vanity or trying to be beautiful; it's also about making sure that your health is in check!

With the help of this book, you'll learn about how to make delicious and nutritious smoothies that will help you lose weight in no time!

What are you waiting for? Start reading this book now and get in the kitchen as soon as you can!

Once again, thank you and enjoy!

Chapter 1: Smoothie Recipes for Breakfast

Here are some smoothies that will surely start your day right so you could go through your day well. Try these healthy smoothies regularly and you'd realize how important it is to drink only the right kind of drinks!

Cannellini Broccoli Smoothie

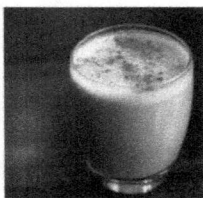

Ingredients:

¼ cup broccoli florets (without the stems)

10 almonds

6 oz Vanilla Non-Fat Greek Yogurt

¼ cup Cannellini beans

1 cup frozen strawberries

¼ tsp cinnamon

¼ tsp flax meal

Directions:

Place each of the ingredients in a blender or food processor then process until smooth.

Then, pour the contents into a glass. Garnish with cinnamon and serve!

Why is it good for you?

This one contains some of the best fat-burning ingredients, such as cinnamon, strawberries, and broccoli. When you burn fats early in the day, you can be sure that it'll be easy for you to do so for the rest of the day, too!

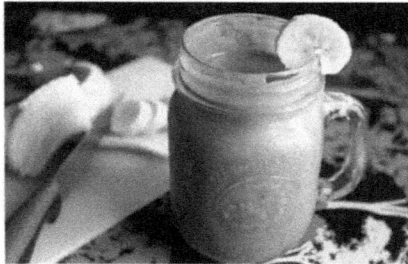

Ingredients:

½ cup non-fat milk

½ cup peanut butter (crunchy or smooth will do)

½ banana

1 Tbsp Whey Chocolate Protein Powder

6 ice cubes

Directions:

Put the banana in the blender, followed by non-fat milk, whey chocolate protein powder, peanut butter, and ice cubes.

Blend until smooth and creamy.

Serve and enjoy!

Why is it good for you?

While you may think that peanut butter is fattening, it's actually a good source of protein, which is also essential when it comes to helping you lose weight. This is also a great pre-workout drink so make sure to consume it before doing your early morning jog!

Flax Apple Surprise

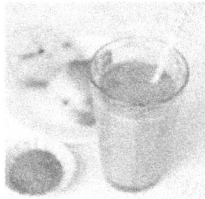

Ingredients:

1 Tbsp ground flax seed

4 almonds, raw

8 oz coconut water

½ scoop protein powder, unsweetened

1 tsp ground cinnamon

1 tsp vanilla extract

Directions:

Place each of the ingredients in a food processor or blender.

Process until smooth or for at least 10 to 15 seconds.

Serve immediately with ice. However, you can also make this overnight so it will already be chilled by the time you drink it in the morning.

Enjoy!

Why is it good for you?

Apples energize you, and when you are energized, your metabolic rate works in such a way that fats are easily burned so you can definitely expect that you'll lose weight!

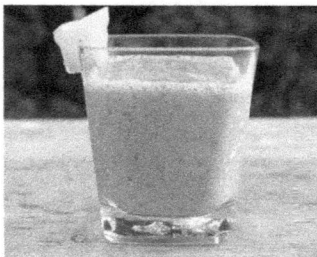

Ingredients:

1 cup kale, packed and chopped

½ cup pineapple, diced

1 banana

1 cup almond milk, unsweetened

½ cup pineapple juice

Directions:

Place kale in the bottom of a blender or food processor.

Add banana, pineapple juice, and almond milk.

Process until smooth, or for at least 15 seconds.

Serve and enjoy!

Why is it good for you?

Pineapples have high fiber content. They cleanse your system and make you feel refreshed and rejuvenated. They enable you to flush out toxins and make room for nutrients!

Kale Berry Smoothie

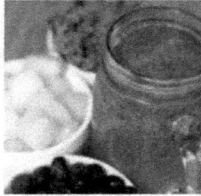

Ingredients:

½ cup pineapple, frozen

½ cup blueberries, frozen

1 Tbsp almond butter

3 oz non-fat Vanilla Greek Yogurt

¾ cup water

1 cup kale

Directions:

Place kale in the bottom of a food processor or blender.

Add blueberries, pineapple, Greek yogurt, and almond butter.

Pour water over the ingredients then process for 15 to 20 seconds or until smooth.

Serve cold and enjoy!

Why is it good for you?

You'll get a lot of protein and calcium from this which is good because they both help in weight loss. Pineapples banish the feelings of bloating and can regulate proper digestion. And, blueberries, aside from being rich in anti-oxidants that can keep you safe from free radicals, are also rich in enzymes that burn belly fat. Plus, it uses water so there are definitely no calories in there. So, you see, you can get most of the nutrients that you need from this one!

Chapter 2: Smoothie Recipes for Lunch

The smoothie recipes in this chapter are those that you can either consume at home, or bring with you to work or wherever it is that you need to go! This way, you won't feel like you're losing energy in the middle of the day and you can keep on doing your responsibilities, too.

Amazing Avocado Smoothie

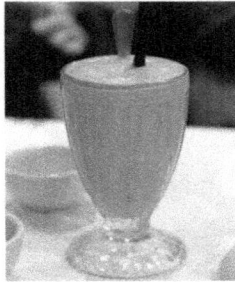

Ingredients:

1 avocado (you may use all of it or cut it in half, if desired)

2 to 4 Tbsp condensed milk, sweetened

½ cup soy milk

Juice of ½ lime

A handful of ice

Directions:

Place avocado in the blender or food processor.

Add lime juice, condensed milk, soy milk, and ice and process for around 20 to 30 seconds or until smooth and creamy,

Serve cold and enjoy!

Why is it good for you?

Avocados contain fat, yes, but they contain the good kind of fat. These reduce LDL or bad cholesterol in your blood and can prevent heart diseases. Avocado is also a good source of dietary fiber so of course, you can expect your body to be detoxified from that and you can expect that you'll lose weight, too! This one can also energize you in the middle of the day—which is truly beneficial.

Majestic Mango Smoothie

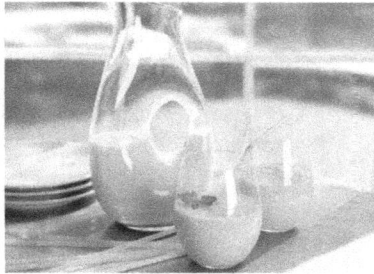

Ingredients:

¼ cup avocado, mashed

¼ cup mango cubes

1 Tbsp sugar

1 Tbsp lime juice

¼ cup fat-free vanilla yogurt

½ cup mango juice

Directions:

Put mango cubes in a blender followed by avocado, lime juice, sugar, vanilla yogurt, and mango juice.

Process until smooth then serve with ice and sliced mangoes, if desired.

Enjoy!

Why is it good for you?

This is full of fiber with very little fat, so you can be sure that it won't add up to your weight. Plus, it has avocado, too, and you know now that avocado does a lot to keep your health in check, which means that this smoothie is something that you really have to make!

Nutty Minty Surprise

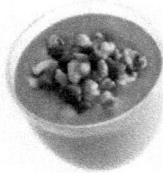

Ingredients:

1 cup almond milk

2 cups fresh spinach

¼ cup rolled oats

2 scoops whey chocolate protein powder

1/8 tsp peppermint extract

1 Tbsp 70% chocolate chips (optional)

1 Tbsp walnuts (optional)

Directions:

Place spinach in the food processor or blender then add rolled oats, protein powder, peppermint extract, and almond milk.

Process for around 15 to 20 seconds or until smooth.

Pour contents into a glass then serve topped with a tablespoon of walnuts or chocolate chips, if desired.

Why is it good for you?

Even just by the smell, you'll already be tempted to try it. What's more, it's amazing because spinach contains dietary fiber that curbs your appetite and regulates digestion. It is also full of Vitamin A that strengthens the body and protects it from intestinal, urinary, and respiratory infections. Aside from that, the Vitamin K content of this smoothie promotes healthy brain function, and strengthens the nervous system as well!

Soy Pumpkin Surprise

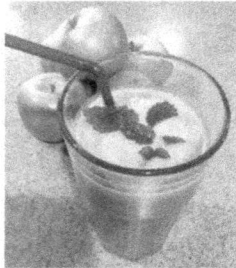

Ingredients:

½ cup canned pumpkin

½ tsp pumpkin spice

½ cup low-fat soy milk

1 Tbsp hot water

3 packs sugar substitute

½ cup cold water

Ice cubes

Directions:

First, make sure that you dissolve the sugar substitute in hot water.

Then, put canned pumpkin, pumpkin spice and soy milk in the blender.

Process it for around 10 seconds, and then stop to add the ice and blend some more until ice is crushed.

Serve immediately and enjoy!

Why is it good for you?

Pumpkin contains no cholesterol—which is not only beneficial for losing weight but can also strengthen your heart and therefore keep heart ailments at bay. Pumpkin also has very low amount of calories and contains a lot of anti-oxidants and vitamins that can protect you against most cancers, plus it also prevents macular degeneration—which makes this smoothie really healthy!

Tofu and Blueberry Smoothie

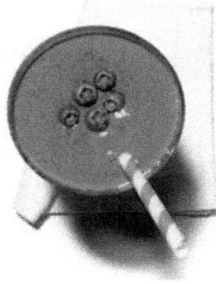

Ingredients:

½ cup silken tofu

1 cup blueberries, frozen

½ cup ice, crushed

½ cup pomegranate juice

1 Tbsp honey or agave nectar

Directions:

Place blueberries in the food processor or blender and then add silken tofu, honey and pomegranate juice.

Blend for at least 5 seconds then add ice and process until smooth.

Serve cold and enjoy!

Why is it good for you?

While this may seem like a weird combination of ingredients, it's actually quite palatable! Again, tofu is a great meat substitute. So, even if you don't eat meat for a certain given time or for a day, you can be sure that you won't lose all the nutrients that you need and that you're still going to be energetic. Blueberries protect you against free radicals and can also promote proper digestion while the Pomegranate Juice enhances digestive processes and cleanses your system because it is full of fiber, the benefits of which have been discussed in the Almond, Pineapple, and Kale Smoothie. This smoothie is an amazing meal replacement for lunch. It's filling but non-fattening!

Best Beet Smoothie

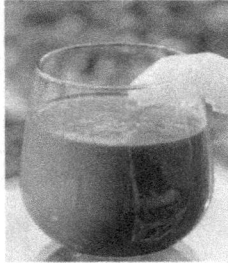

Ingredients:

1 small can of beets

3 ice cubes

1 cup tofu

Directions:

Place beets in the blender or food processor.

Add tofu and ice cubes and process until smooth and creamy.

Serve cold and enjoy! If you're bringing it with you to the office, make sure to keep it in the refrigerator before consuming.

Why is it good for you?

Beets are some of the most nutritious foods on the planet. They contain a lot of antioxidants, as well as fiber and potassium that are all essential for keeping your digestive processes in check and making sure that your body systems are all working properly. Best of all, they also help you absorb nutrients from most of the things you eat, too! Tofu has always been a popular meat substitute, so even if you do not eat meat, you can expect that you'll feel healthy and that you won't lose energy.

Cheesy Banana Smoothie

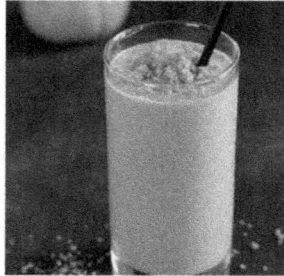

Ingredients:

½ cup vanilla almond milk, unsweetened

1 frozen banana

¼ cup low-fat cottage cheese

½ cup Vanilla Greek Yogurt

2 cinnamon cream cheese wedges

Directions:

Put banana in the food processor then add cottage cheese, cheese wedges and Greek Yogurt.

Pour vanilla almond milk and pulse until smooth and creamy.

Serve with extra cheese crumbs, if desired.

Enjoy!

Why is it good for you?

Cheese is not entirely bad, especially when you take the lowofat varieties in small amounts. There are good kinds of cheese, such as cottage cheese that contain loads of calcium without making you fat. Aside from that, it also adds a lot of flavor to your smoothie.

Bananas, on the other hand are also full of fiber and potassium that regulate digestive processes so you could easily burn fat and absorb nutrients that are better for you!

Chapter 3: Smoothie Recipes for Dinner

When it comes to making smoothie recipes for dinner, it's important that you choose greens, fruits, and other ingredients that will not add up to your body fat. After all, metabolism is naturally slow at night so you have to make sure that your body won't have a hard time digesting what you take. And these recipes are surely going to end your day right because you get to cut on your fat consumption.

Cheery Cherry Smoothie

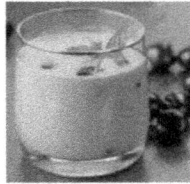

Ingredients:

¾ cup cranberry juice

15 very ripe fresh or canned cherries, pitted

¼ tsp almond extract

2 scoops frozen vanilla yogurt

Extra cranberries, for garnish (optional)

Directions:

Put cherries in the food processor or blender then add vanilla yogurt, almond extract, and cranberry juice.

Process until smooth.

Garnish with extra cranberries, if desired.

Serve and enjoy!

Why is it good for you?

Cranberries are good for the heart, and when your heart is healthy, you know that you're healthy, too! Plus they also contain loads of Vitamin C that can protect your body against most diseases so you could easily burn fat. They are also linked to cancer prevention.

Cherries, meanwhile, are great to consume at night because they keep your mind and body relaxed. They enhance metabolism, too, so of course, you can easily burn fat and say goodbye to calories!

Fruity Spinach Surprise

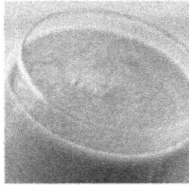

Ingredients:

2 cups spinach

1 banana, peeled and chopped

1 orange, peeled and segmented

½ cup Plain Greek Yogurt

2 cups Spinach

1 cup ice

Directions:

Place spinach, oranges, and banana into your blender then process for around 30 seconds.

Then, stop and add the ice and yogurt and work on it again until it's smooth.

Serve cold and enjoy!

Why is it good for you?

Spinach is one of the healthiest greens in the world. It regulates digestive processes, makes it easy for your body to absorb nutrients, and can also strengthen your immune system—no wonder Popeye loves it so much!

Oranges and Banana have fiber that cleanse the body and can protect you against respiratory diseases so they're great for you, too. Now, you won't have a hard time digesting this nutritious food!

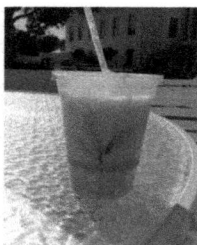

Ingredients:

A pinch of cayenne pepper

1 Tbsp ginger, grated finely

1 Tbsp fresh lemon juice

½ cup avocado

6 oz carrot juice

¼ cup water

Directions:

Place avocado in the blender then add ginger, cayenne pepper, lemon juice and carrot juice before adding water.

Process for around 15 to 20 seconds or until smooth.

Serve cold and enjoy!

Why is it good for you?

Spices contain Capsaicin. Capsaicin is beneficial because it boosts your metabolism and curbs your appetite. This is the reason why there are times when after you eat some spicy food, you feel like you're already full. Plus, what's great about this smoothie is that it also soothes sore muscles, mostly because of ginger. It may be a surprising mix, but it's definitely healthy and delicious!

Kefir Herb Mix

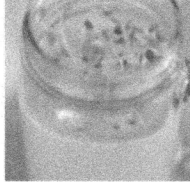

Ingredients:

9 oz kefir

3 to 4 Tbsp chopped mix herbs of your choice

2 Tbsp bean sprouts

White pepper

Salt

½ Tbsp honey

2 Tbsp lemon juice

Directions:

Make sure that you have washed the bean sprouts thoroughly before using them.

Then, put herbs in the food processor or blender.

Add kefir, honey, salt, pepper, and lemon juice.

Blend until smooth or for around 15 to 20 seconds.

Add more pepper or salt, to taste, then blend again.

Garnish with sprouts, if desired.

Enjoy!

Why is it good for you?

This is another unusual mix of ingredients, especially for a smoothie, but it's great in the sense that kefir relaxes the nervous system. When you are relaxed and when you're not stressed out, you do not think about eating more especially if you are already full. It's also full of amino acids that protect you against most diseases and it can also regulate digestive processes as well.

Healthy Piña Colada

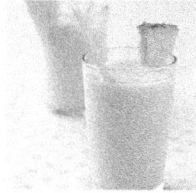

Ingredients:

½ cup pineapple

½ cup coconut water

½ cup almond milk, unsweetened

1 Tbsp coconut, shredded

1 tsp honey

¼ tsp vanilla extract

½ cup ice

Directions:

Put pineapple in the blender.

Add shredded coconut, vanilla extract, honey, almond milk, and coconut water.

Blend for around 10 to 15 seconds.

Add ice and blend for another 10 seconds.

Serve immediately and enjoy.

Why is it good for you?

Who says that Pina Coladas are just for parties and cannot be healthy? This version is something that you'll want to make because it is full of fiber that can cleanse and rejuvenate your system. Plus, the mixture of almond milk and water is healthy and filling, too, without adding calories to your system. It's one of the best that you can make!

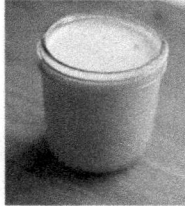

Ingredients:

½ cup unsalted cashew nuts, chopped coarsely

¼ cup honey

4 cups orange juice

4 cups water

Directions:

Put cashew nuts in the food processor or blender.

Add honey and orange juice then pour water and process for 10 to 15 seconds or until creamy and smooth.

Serve cold and enjoy!

Why is it good for you?

The best thing about this smoothie is that it contains a lot of dietary fiber, mainly because of the cashews. They help out in weight management, especially when consumed at least once or twice a week. Orange and honey give this smoothie a tasty flavor that's sure to make your taste buds happy!

Buttery Mango Smoothie

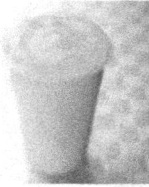

Ingredients:

½ cup buttermilk

1 cup mango, peeled, pitted, and chopped

½ tsp lemon juice

1 tsp honey

1/3 cup ice, crushed

¼ tsp lemon peel, grated

Strawberries, for garnish (optional)

Directions:

Put mango in the blender, followed by honey, buttermilk, lemon peel, and lemon juice.

Process for 10 seconds.

Add crushed ice then process for 10 seconds more or until smooth.

Garnish with strawberries, if desired.

Serve and enjoy!

Why is it good for you?

Ignore the name: Buttermilk is good for you because it contains no fat and has a lot of calcium which is essential to help you grow properly. Mango and Buttermilk contains a lot of vitamins and minerals such as Riboflavin, Vitamin B12, and Phosphorus that regulate digestion, enhance metabolism, and detoxify your body.

Crazy Good Cantaloupe

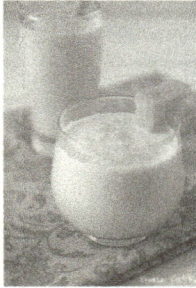

Ingredients:

½ cup Plain Greek Yogurt

½ cantaloupe, seeded and then chopped roughly

3 ice cubes

1 Tbsp honey

Directions:

Place cantaloupe in the blender then add honey, Greek Yogurt, and ice cubes.

Process for around 15 to 20 seconds then serve and enjoy!

Why is it good for you?

Cantaloupe is considered as a superfood because it can boost your metabolism in more ways than one. It is composed of 89% water so you know that it's actually non-fattening and that it does a lot to help you lose weight. Honey adds a lot of flavor into this, making it a really enjoyable drink!

Sage and Passion Fruit Surprise

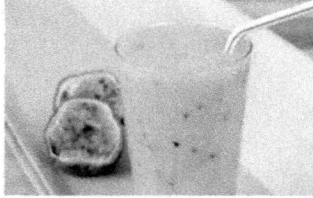

Ingredients:

1 small mango, peeled, pitted, and chopped

2 passion fruit

4 fresh sage leaves, chopped roughly

2 cups milk

1 small banana, peeled and chopped

Directions:

First, make sure that you cut the passion fruit into two. Scrape the seeds and pulp and put them in a liquidizer so you could still make use of them for this smoothie. You can also just heat the seeds and get the juice through a sieve.

Then, pour the contents into a blender and add banana, sage leaves, and mango.

Pour 2 cups of milk then process until smooth.

Serve cold and enjoy!

Why is it good for you?

Passion Fruit is very beneficial because it is a great source of potassium, dietary fiber, sterols, and Vitamins A and C that can lower bad cholesterol levels and can also help the body relax so appetite can be curbed and digestive processes will be regulated and that's why it's recommended that you drink this for dinner or just shortly before going to bed. This way, it can help you sleep soundly, too!

Chapter 4: Smoothie Recipes for Snacks

Make snack time valuable and fun by drinking smoothies that won't add up to your weight. In this chapter, you'll learn how to make some of them. Enjoy them by yourself, or serve them to your family and friends while watching movies or just spending time with one another.

The Sweet Potato Shake

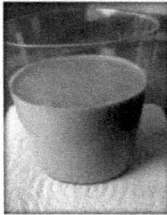

Ingredients:

½ cup sweet potato, peeled, cooked and diced

1 Tbsp cinnamon whey protein powder

3 ice cubes

1 cup vanilla almond milk

Directions:

Put sweet potato in the blender.

Add vanilla almond milk and cinnamon whey protein powder and blend for 10 seconds.

Add ice and blend for another 10 seconds.

Serve and enjoy!

Why is it good for you?

This sounds weird but it's actually very beneficial because sweet potatoes and cinnamon protein powder can replenish glycogen stores in your body. This means that after drinking this smoothie, you'll feel all the more energized, especially if you choose to drink this after working out. That makes it a great accompaniment to your snack periods because you'll be able to do more once you are energized and so you will be able to burn fat!

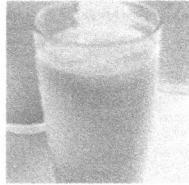

Ingredients:

1 tsp ginseng root, sliced (if this is not available, you can use ginseng powder instead)

1 tsp white tea leaves (you can also use a bag of white tea)

2 pineapple rings, chopped

5 oz orange juice, freshly squeezed

1 small honeydew melon wedge, peeled, seeded, and chopped

8 oz hot water

Directions:

First, put the tea leaves or white tea bag in a pitcher.

Add ginseng to the pitcher, followed by hot water then let it brew for around 2 to 3 minutes. If you're using ginseng root and tea leaves, make sure that you do not forget to strain after.

Put some ice cubes to the pitcher so the tea will easily cool down.

Then, put pineapple and melon on the blender.

Add orange juice and white tea.

Process for around 15 seconds or until smooth.

Serve and enjoy!

Why is it good for you?

White tea is actually the least processed tea of all, which means that it basically has no preservatives and can boost your metabolic rate the right way. It also contains a lot of antioxidants that keep you safe from free radicals and allow you to look fresh and healthy! This way, you do not only lose weight, you can also be sure that you stay radiant and young-looking, too!

The Healthy Minty Mojito

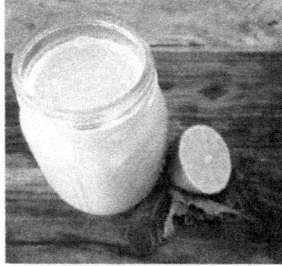

Ingredients:

2 Tbsp hemp seeds

1 cup coconut water

2 Tbsp lime juice, freshly squeezed

½ to 1 tsp spirulina

A handful of fresh mint leaves

2 dates, pitted

1 frozen banana

½ avocado

Directions:

Place the avocado in the food processor or blender, then add banana, dates, mint leaves, spirulina, hemp seeds, and lime juice.

Add coconut water then process for around 15 to 20 seconds or until smooth.

Serve cold and enjoy!

Why is it good for you?

Who says that a Mojito can't be healthy? This one contains avocado, that can reduce bad cholesterol in your blood plus it also has spirulina, an algae that contains B-Vitamins and protein that turn fat into energy, so they can be burned and yet, you can still be able to use them for good! This mojito will also help you absorb only the nutrients that you need!

Date, Almond, and Chocolate Smoothie

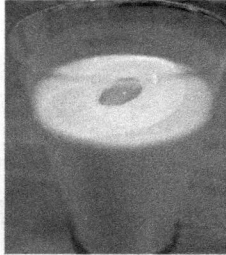

Ingredients:

½ cup dates, pitted

¼ cup almonds

½ cup boiling water

¼ cup cocoa powder

3 ice cubes

½ cup silken tofu

Directions:

Put cocoa, almonds, and dates in the blender together with hot water and just let the mixture stay there for around 10 minutes without blending.

Then, add tofu and ice and process for around 15 to 20 seconds or until smooth and creamy.

Serve cold and enjoy!

You may also serve this with extra chopped dates on top, if desired.

Why is it good for you?

While dates may contain some calories, what's great is that they also contain the right amount of nutrients that are higher than calories so you know that it won't add up to your weight. It's also refreshing and relaxing which can drive stress away!

Carrot and Grapefruit Smoothie

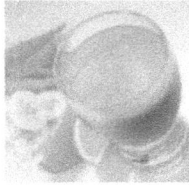

Ingredients:

3 cups water

3 carrots, peeled and chopped coarsely

½ tsp powdered ginger

1 ½ Tbsp honey

4 cups grapefruit juice, unsweetened

Directions:

First, cook the carrots in a pan with ½ cup water. Do this for around 10 minutes in low heat.

Then, drain and keep the cooking liquid from the carrots.

Puree the carrots in a blender then add ginger, grapefruit juice, honey, and the rest of the water.

Blend until frothy.

Serve cold and enjoy!

Why is it good for you?

Grapefruit is a big part of most diets because it contains a lot of water and no calories that can definitely aid in weight loss. What's more, it can also keep you safe from common colds and flu—especially when mixed with carrots!

Amazing Apple Smoothie

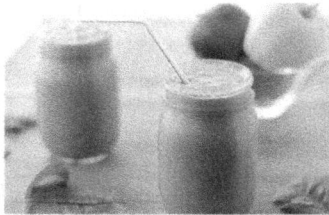

Ingredients:

1 apple, sliced (green or red will do)

¼ cup cashews

½ frozen banana

2 dates, pitted

1 scoop hemp protein

1 tsp apple pie spice

1 cup almond milk

3 ice cubes

Directions:

Put the apple slices in the food processor or blender then add banana, cashews, dates, apple pie spice, hemp protein, and ice cubes.

Process for around 20 to 30 seconds or until smooth.

Serve cold and enjoy!

Why is it good for you?

This smoothie contains a lot of protein and fatty acids that enhance metabolism and cleanse your system so you'd feel healthy and rejuvenated. Apples energize you while it burns your calories away so it's great, especially for an all-nighter. It's definitely a great smoothie snack so you have to try it out!

Flax and Prune Smoothie

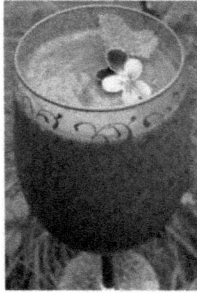

Ingredients:

5 prunes, pitted

1 banana, peeled and chopped

1 Tbsp pure flax oil

1 cup plain low-fat yogurt

¼ cup orange juice

Directions:

Put prunes, banana, flax oil, yogurt, and orange juice in the blender.

Blend for around 15 seconds or until smooth.

Serve and enjoy!

Why is it good for you?

Before you roll your eyes as to how this will taste like, you do have to give it a try first. This smoothie is beneficial because it is rich in fiber which can regulate digestive processes and enhance metabolism. It's also rich in Omega-3 which can keep your heart young and healthy!

Chapter 5: Smoothie Recipes for Dessert

And of course, you have to make some smoothies that are perfect for desserts, too! A lot of people connect desserts to fatty foods but contrary to popular belief, you can actually make smoothie desserts that are delicious but won't let you pack on the pounds! Here are some of them.

Tiramisu for Health Buffs

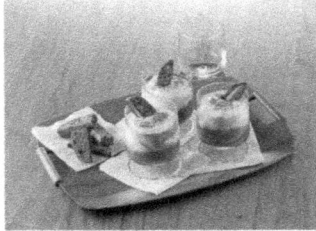

Ingredients:

2 Tbsp low fat Plain-Greek Yogurt

1/3 cup part-skim ricotta cheese

1 tsp ground flaxseed

1 scoop chocolate whey protein powder

3 ice cubes

1 Tbsp finely ground coffee

Directions:

Place ricotta cheese, chocolate whey protein powder, flaxseed, yogurt, and ground coffee in a blender.

Process for 10 to 15 seconds or until creamy.

Add ice cubes then blend for 10 seconds more or until frothy.

Serve cold and enjoy!

Why is it good for you?

This one may be creamy and chocolaty but it actually contains very few calories plus it also has ricotta, which makes it rich in protein that is extremely good for you! This way, calories will be burned and you'll still savor the delicious taste of this.

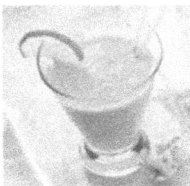

Ingredients:

1 ripe banana, sliced

1 pack key lime pie yogurt

1 Tbsp lime juice

½ cup 2% milk

1 cup vanilla frozen yogurt

¼ tsp lemon lime flavored soft drink

Directions:

Place bananas in the blender, followed by lime pie yogurt, vanilla yogurt, lime juice, milk, and lemon lime soft drink.

Blend on high until smooth.

Serve cold and enjoy!

Why is it good for you?

Don't worry about the minimal soft drink content. It's lime, after all, so it has lots of Vitamin C. It's also very beneficial because of bananas that contain lots of Potassium. This has some fiber, too, so your body will be cleansed and you'll be able to burn some fat.

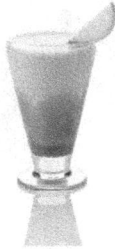

Ingredients:

½ cup low-fat vanilla ice cream

1 cup apple cider

1 Tbsp caramel sauce

3 ice cubes

½ tsp cinnamon

Directions:

Place vanilla ice cream in the blender then add caramel sauce, cinnamon, apple cider and ice cubes.

Blend on high until smooth and creamy.

Serve immediately and enjoy!

Why is it good for you?

Apple Cider has long been known to have fat-burning capabilities and this time, you won't have a hard time consuming it because it's turned into a delicious smoothie! This also contains lots of Vitamin C and Potassium that your body needs!

Pear and Ginger Smoothie

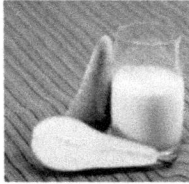

Ingredients:

1 ¼ cups ginger ice cream

1 ripe pear, cored and chopped

2 ginger cookies, crumbled

3 Tbsp heavy whipping cream

Directions:

Put pear in the blender.

Add whipping cream and ginger ice cream.

Process for at least 45 to 50 seconds or until frothy.

Serve immediately and enjoy!

Why is it good for you?

This one is a bit spicy, which is good because it contains Capsaicin that burns body fat fast. At the same time, it also has pear which contains a lct of water and no calories so you can expect that you'll definitely lose weight!

Creamy Peach Smoothie

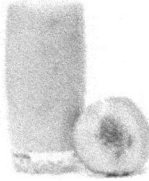

Ingredients:

½ cup whole milk

½ can peach halves, juice intact

3 Tbsp peach liquor

1 ½ scoops vanilla ice cream

¼ cup half and half

1 scoop peach ice cream

½ cup peach slices

Directions:

First, place the peach halves in the blender together with ¼ cup juice.

Process until smooth then place some of the puree in a pitcher. Set it aside.

Add ice cream, half and half, milk, and peach liquor then process for around 15 seconds or until smooth.

Serve with the rest of the ice cream and peach slices and enjoy!

Why is it good for you?

This one is the liquefied version of your classic peaches and cream. It's tasty and filling and it does not pack on the pounds because peaches also contain loads of water. They have lots of Vitamin C, too, so your immune system would be given a boost and you'll be protected against most diseases!

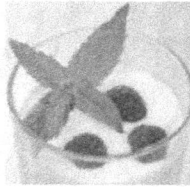

Ingredients:

1 cup fresh or frozen raspberries

8 fresh mint leaves

2 scoops vanilla frozen yogurt

Sugar, to taste

½ cup low-fat milk

Extra raspberries and mint leaves, for garnish (optional)

Directions:

Place milk and mint leaves in the blender.

Blend until smooth or until mints have been chopped finely.

Serve garnished with mint leaves or raspberries, if desired.

Enjoy!

Why is it good for you?

Mint can produce enzymes that can hasten digestion so you'll definitely be able to lose weight. It's the reason why a lot of people chew gum after eating! Raspberries are full of antioxidants so you'll be safe from free radicals.

The Healthy Black Forest

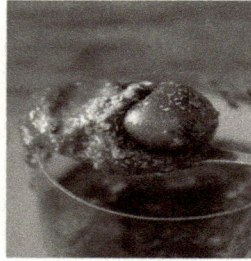

Ingredients:

½ frozen banana

2 scoops hemp smoothie protein powder

¼ cup almond milk, unsweetened

1 Tbsp raw cocoa powder

½ cup frozen cherries, pitted

1 tsp dark chocolate shavings, for garnish (optional)

4 ice cubes

Directions:

Put banana, cherries, cocoa powder, protein powder, and ice in a blender.

Blend on high until creamy.

Serve topped with dark chocolate servings, if desired.

Enjoy!

Why is it good for you?

This one maybe sweet but it's also full of protein and it definitely will not make you gain weight, mostly because cocoa, dark chocolate, and hemp are used. Cherries regulate digestion and are full of antioxidants plus dark chocolate actually curbs your appetite so you won't feel hungry all the time. It's one dessert that you definitely won't forget.

Chapter 6: Final Reminders

Now that you have made the recipes mentioned in this book, what's next? Well, you could create your own recipes, too.

To make sure that the recipes you'll make will help you burn fat and won't make you gain weight, here are some tips that you have to keep in mind:

1. **Fresh over Frozen.** Of course, you may not always have fresh fruits or vegetables around and there are times when you keep frozen ones in the fridges, but as much as possible, go for fresh. Why? Simply because they are more nutritious and they have not been processed. If you want to make the most out of your ingredients, going fresh is the way.

2. **Greens are your best friend.** While there are a couple of ingredients that you can use, it would be a good idea to make greens as your base, especially during lunch or dinner. They make the smoothies more filling and they can detoxify the body. Plus, using greens always adds a different bit of flavor to your drinks so you have to have them around as much as you can.

3. **It would be good to process the greens first.** You can either place them first in the blender or process them first before mixing them with the rest of the ingredients. This way, you can be sure that those vegetables won't be chunky and you won't have a hard time digesting them.

4. **Tea boosts nutrition.** Instead of always relying on milk or water, why not go for tea? It can enhance metabolism, especially if you use White or Green Tea, plus they make your smoothies more flavorful, too!

5. **Make use of super foods.** Super foods can make your smoothies healthier and can boost metabolism in more ways than one. The best ones that you can use include coconut oil, bee pollen, goji berries, cacao, maca, spirulina, acai berries and hemp seeds.

6. **Blend seeds.** It's a good thing that you can make smoothies with the use of blenders and food processors because you can thoroughly crush seeds so you can get their flavors and you'll be able to benefit from them, too. Flaxseed and Chia Seeds are some of the best that you could try.

7. **Dates can work as sweeteners.** Instead of adding sugar or stevia, or other artificial sweeteners, you can use dates to sweeten your smoothies. It would be nice to have them pitted first then soak them for around 8 to 12 hours or overnight before mixing them with the rest of your ingredients. This is especially helpful during cold, winter months when fruits and vegetables aren't as tasty as you want them to be.

8. **Make use of Protein.** You can get a lot of protein from fish and eggs but of course, you really cannot blend those things because they might make the

smoothies a bit crazy for you. However, you can make use of Protein Powder so you can be sure that you'll get the right amount of protein that you need and that you'll be able to burn fat faster. There are a couple of flavors to choose from, too, so you won't get bored!

9. **Using spices are helpful, too.** Spices contain capsaicin so they are able to burn fat and amp up the taste of your smoothies. When the smoothies are tasty, you won't be bored and so you will keep on making various kinds of smoothies that will help you lose weight. The best spices that you can use include cayenne, nutmeg, cinnamon, and ginger.

10. **And, use liquids.** Spring or Filtered water contains no calories and can hydrate you. Coconut Water has a lot of electrolytes that can energize you, while almond, soy milk, or fresh fruit juice thicken the smoothie and make it more flavorful. Liquids can also make the smoothies easier to drink so the experience will really be smooth!

Remember, these smoothies can help you get in tip-top shape so you have to make sure that you know how to make them. Keep these tips in mind and you'll be able to create the most flavorful and nutritious smoothies that will help you lose weight!

Conclusion

Thank you for reading this book!

I hope this book was able to help you create enticing and nutritious smoothies that will help you burn fat and lose weight.

Finally, if you enjoyed this book, please take time to post a review. It will be greatly appreciated.

www.ingramcontent.com/pod-product-compliance
Lightning Source LLC
Chambersburg PA
CBHW030305030426
42337CB00012B/598